Table of Contents

The Brain Revival Plan: Steps to Reclaim and Enhance Your Mind
© Copyright 2024 **Nicole Yeates**

ISBN: 978-0-646-70626-9

Dedication

To my incredible mother, whose unwavering love and belief in me, even when the medical world saw only darkness, gave me the strength to defy the odds. Though you are no longer here on this earth, I know you continue to guide me, and I feel your presence in every step I take.

Since your passing, I believe you sent me a sign that true love can come into our lives more than once. To John, who came into my life and restored my faith in love. Thank you for your boundless support, love, and trust in my purpose. Your patience and perseverance mean more to me than words can express, especially with my workaholic tendencies.

This book is for both of you - my heart, strength, and inspiration.

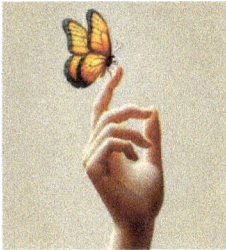

INTRODUCTION

"Your brain is the architect of your reality; nurture it and watch your world transform."

Nicole Yeates

When my mother was told I'd never regain the full function of my brain after a severe traumatic injury on 19 June 1987, it felt like a life sentence. But deep inside, I refused to accept that fate. I hoped there had to be a way to survive and thrive. I held on to this hope. My journey from a prognosis of expected death or life in a vegetative state to a life full of purpose and potential was not easy, but it was possible because I learned how to work with my brain rather than against it.

This book is for those who find themselves at a crossroads, wondering how to move forward when their brain is not working right. This can be after trauma, unexpected life changes, such as acquired injury, mental illness, neurodiversity, or any of the myriads of events that can keep us stuck.

If you know your brain holds the key to your future but aren't sure how to unlock your potential, this book is for you! It's for anyone ready to take steps to promote healing and optimise brain health for the long term.

If you have watched your loved ones slow, devastating pathway through Alzheimer's Disease or any type of Dementia, and you want to reduce your risks of losing your own mind.... keep reading.

In the following pages, you'll find a roadmap to understanding your brain, reviewing its current state, and crafting a personalised plan to optimise it.

Whether you're just beginning your journey or are further along the path, this guide will provide you with the tools and strategies to discover the new you - stronger, more focused, and more resilient than ever before.

Brain change takes consistency and persistency!

Let's embark on this journey together. The new you is waiting to be discovered, and it all starts with your brain.

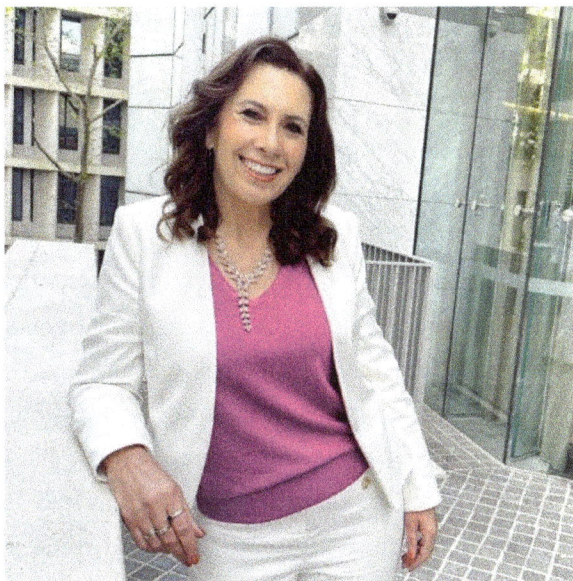

GET**Brain**FIT

CHAPTER 1: What is Brain Health?

Your brain is a muscle to be exercised regularly, just like your body!

Brain health means how well your brain works in thinking, feeling, behaving, and overall wellness. It includes keeping the brain's structure healthy, ensuring it works smoothly, and handling new challenges, stress, and injuries. Like your body, your brain needs regular care and attention to keep it working at its best.

Why is Brain Health Important?

The brain is the control centre of your entire body. It regulates everything from basic functions like breathing and heart rate to complex processes like decision-making, memory, and emotional regulation. When your brain is healthy, you are more likely to experience clear thinking, emotional balance, effective problem-solving, and resilience in the face of stress. Conversely, poor brain health can lead to cognitive decline, emotional instability, and behavioral issues that can significantly impact your quality of life. When our brain works right, we work right!

Did you know that our brain shrinks by an average of 5% per decade after the age of 40? (Amen 2018).

That's right! That is the brain's natural aging progression. However, it does not have to be that way if we are building our brain reserves over our lifetime!

The Impact of Brain Health on Life

Cognition: Brain health affects your cognitive abilities, including memory, attention, reasoning, and learning. A well-nurtured brain can enhance your ability to process information, retain knowledge, and apply it effectively in your daily life. Cognitive sharpness is crucial not just for academic or professional success, but also for making informed decisions and navigating life's challenges. We make better decisions with a healthy brain!

Emotion: Emotional health is closely tied to brain health. The brain regulates mood, stress responses, and emotional resilience. When your brain is functioning optimally, you are better equipped to manage stress, avoid burnout, and maintain a positive outlook on life. Conversely, poor brain health can lead to anxiety, depression, and emotional volatility.

So why is brain health rarely considered in pathways to improved mental health?

Behaviour: Your behaviour reflects your brain's health. A healthy brain supports self-control, goal-directed behavior, and forming and maintaining healthy habits. It helps you resist impulsive actions, make thought-out decisions, and stay motivated toward your goals. Poor brain health, on the other hand, can lead to impulsivity, lack of focus, and difficulty sticking to positive routines.

Well-being: Overall well-being is deeply connected to the state of your brain. A healthy brain contributes to a sense of purpose, fulfillment, and contentment. It enables you to form meaningful relationships, pursue your passions, and live a life aligned with your values. By contrast, a brain not cared for can lead to disconnection, dissatisfaction, and a lack of fulfillment.

How Brain Health Affects Various Aspects of Life

Work and Productivity: A healthy brain enhances one's ability to focus, stay organised, and think creatively, leading to greater productivity and success in professional life.

Relationships: Emotional regulation and empathy, both governed by brain health, are essential for forming and maintaining healthy relationships. A well-functioning brain helps you connect with others, understand their perspectives, and communicate effectively.

Physical Health: The brain is linked to physical health. Research has clearly shown that chronic stress can cause physical illnesses such as high blood pressure, while positive mental health can boost immune function and overall vitality.

Personal Growth: A healthy brain is the foundation for personal growth. It allows you to set and achieve goals, adapt to change, and continuously improve yourself. Brain health is key to your success, whether learning a new skill, overcoming a challenge, or striving for personal excellence.

In The Brain Revival Plan: Steps to Reclaim and Enhance Your Mind, we will explore practical strategies for enhancing brain health, reclaiming your cognitive abilities, and revitalising your life.

Whether you've experienced a brain injury, cognitive decline or want to optimise your mental performance to remember more, focus better and be more productive, this guide will provide you with the tools to achieve your goals and live a fulfilling, empowered life.

Reducing Risks: The incidence of Alzheimer's Disease (a type of Dementia) is on the rise. The most significant factor contributing to this is that people are living longer.

Alzheimer's is primarily an age-related condition, with most cases occurring in people over 65 (although it can occur earlier than this). As life expectancy increases globally, the number of older adults who are at higher risk for Alzheimer's also increases, leading to more cases of this disease (Alzheimer's Association, 2024).

In Australia, approximately 1 in 12 people aged 65 and over are living with Dementia, and this prevalence rises to 2 in 5 among those aged 90 and over (Australian Government Department of Health and Aged Care, 2023).

Modern lifestyle factors, such as poor diet, lack of physical activity, smoking, high blood pressure and increased stress, are just some of the things that have been linked to a higher risk of developing Alzheimer's. These factors can contribute to conditions like obesity, diabetes, and heart disease, which are known to increase the risk of cognitive decline and Alzheimer's disease (Amen Clinics, 2024)

Certain chronic health conditions, particularly cardiovascular diseases, high blood pressure, diabetes, and obesity, have been linked to Alzheimer's. These conditions affect blood flow to the brain and contribute to the buildup of harmful proteins (such as amyloid plaques) associated with Alzheimer's.

Exposure to environmental toxins and pollutants may also play a role in increasing Alzheimer's risk. Some studies suggest that air pollution, heavy metals, and pesticides could damage brain health and contribute to cognitive decline. Sedentary lifestyles, high levels of processed foods, and poor sleep habits also exacerbate risk factors.

While age is the biggest risk factor, genetics also play a role. Individuals with a family history of Alzheimer's are more likely to develop the disease. In particular, carrying certain genetic variants like the APOE-e4 gene increases the likelihood of developing Alzheimer's (National Institute on Aging, n.d.).

Lack of mental stimulation, social isolation, and not engaging in activities that challenge the brain can also increase the risk of Alzheimer's. Cognitive decline is more likely in individuals who are not mentally active throughout their lives. (Livingston, G., et al. 2020).

Preventive measures, such as promoting healthy brain habits and early intervention, may help reduce the impact of this growing health issue.

CHAPTER 2: Neuroplasticity: The Brain's Power to Change and Adapt

Neuroplasticity is the brain's incredible ability to reorganise itself by forming new neural connections at any age throughout life. This allows our brain to adapt to new experiences, learn new skills, and recover from brain damage. Neuroplasticity is the foundation of all learning and memory. It will enable us to grow mentally, emotionally, and intellectually, continually shaping our minds based on our experiences, thoughts, and actions (Psychology Today, n.d).

How Neuroplasticity Works

Formation of New Neurons and Connections: Not that long ago, neuroscientists believed that our brain was fixed, like the concrete under our feet. Unchangeable, unadaptable. They believed that once we reached adulthood, we were stuck with the brain we've got!

Neurogenesis is one of the most exciting aspects of neuroplasticity - the process by which new neurons are formed in the brain. This typically occurs in specific brain areas, such as the hippocampus, which is involved in memory and learning. Alongside neurogenesis, the brain continuously forms new synaptic connections. These communication links between neurons are based on experiences and knowledge. For instance, when you learn a new skill or piece of information, your brain strengthens the connections between activated neurons, making it easier to recall or perform that skill in the future (IBE–UNESCO, n.d.).

Strengthening and Weakening of Existing Connections: Neuroplasticity also involves strengthening frequently used neural pathways and weakening less used ones, a concept known as "synaptic pruning." Remember the old saying, *'If you don't use it, you lose it'*?

This is similar to how a well-trodden path through a forest becomes easier to walk on, while a rarely used path becomes overgrown and difficult to navigate. For example, if you practice a musical instrument regularly, the neural connections related to that skill will strengthen, improving proficiency. Conversely, if you stop practicing, those connections may weaken over time, making the skill more difficult to pick up again when you feel in the mood to play that instrument.

Reorganisation and Compensation:
Neuroplasticity allows different brain regions to reorganise and compensate for damage. For

example, if a specific brain area responsible for a particular function is injured, nearby areas can often adapt to take over that function. This is particularly important in recovery from strokes or traumatic brain injuries, where rehabilitation efforts focus on retraining the brain to maximise function.

When I woke up from my deep coma, I was unable to see, walk, talk, smell, or move any part of my body. My sight came back first, then I gained limited movement of one arm. With regular physical therapy from Physiotherapists and massage from family and friends, I slowly gained more movement. Old neural pathways started to awaken with regular practice and rehabilitation.

Neuroplasticity as the Basis for Mind Power
Neuroplasticity is the scientific foundation of what we often call "mind power" - the ability to use your mental faculties to influence your reality and achieve your desired outcomes. Because the brain is adaptable, you have the power to change your thoughts, behaviours, and emotions in ways that can dramatically alter your life. Whether you want to break a bad habit, develop a new skill, or overcome a personal challenge, harnessing the principles of neuroplasticity allows you to reshape your brain and, consequently, your reality.

For instance, by consistently visualising success, engaging in positive self-talk, and practicing mental rehearsal, you can strengthen the neural networks associated with confidence and goal achievement. Over time, this can lead to real-world changes in behaviour, increased resilience, and greater success.

During my rehabilitation following my severe traumatic brain injury, I was fortunate enough to be guided through a visualisation process under deep meditation with my psychologist at the time. Utilising this theta state (a relaxed and suggestible brain state, perfect for reprogramming beliefs) provided an empowering resource to heal my brain, and it worked!

Enhancing or Hindering Neuroplasticity

While neuroplasticity is a powerful tool, its effectiveness can be influenced by several factors:

Age: While neuroplasticity is most pronounced during childhood, it continues throughout life. However, the rate of neurogenesis and the brain's ability to reorganise tend to decrease with age. Nonetheless, adults can still benefit greatly from engaging in activities stimulating neuroplasticity, such as learning new skills, exercising, and maintaining an active social life.

Genetics: Some of us may have a genetic predisposition that enhances or hinders their brain's plasticity. However, genes are not destiny. Even those with less favorable genetics can improve their brain's plasticity through lifestyle choices.

Environment: A stimulating environment rich in learning opportunities, social interaction, and physical activity can significantly enhance neuroplasticity. Alternatively, a deprived or stressful environment can hinder it, reducing cognitive and emotional capacity.

Lifestyle: Regular physical exercise, a balanced diet, sufficient sleep, and stress management support neuroplasticity. Physical activity, in particular, increases blood flow to the brain and promotes neurogenesis.

Mindset: A growth mindset is the belief that abilities and intelligence can be developed, and this fosters neuroplasticity. People with a growth mindset are more likely to see barriers as challenges, learn from mistakes, and persist in the face of setbacks, all of which contribute to stronger and more resilient neural networks.

By understanding and leveraging the principles of neuroplasticity, you can unlock your brain's potential, overcome barriers, and move closer to achieving your desired outcomes. Neuroplasticity is one of the main keys to making it happen, whether recovering from an injury, enhancing your mental faculties, or striving to reach new personal or professional goals.

CHAPTER 3: Rewiring For Success - Turning Mindset into Action

The Difference Between a Fixed Mindset and Growth Mindset

American psychologist Dr. Carol Dweck created the terms "fixed" and "growth" mindsets to explain different, primarily subconscious mindsets.

When you have a fixed mindset, you believe your abilities, intelligence, and talents are static traits that cannot be changed or improved. These people often view challenges as threats to their self-worth, avoid complex tasks, and believe that effort is fruitless if you lack natural talent. This mindset can lead to fear of failure, fear of taking risks, and a tendency to give up easily when obstacles occur.

If you have a growth mindset, you are more likely to believe that your abilities and intelligence can be developed through effort, feedback, and learning. Those with a growth mindset see challenges as opportunities for growth, view effort as a necessary part of success, and are likelier to persist in facing difficulties. Having a growth mindset enables an understanding that learning and improvement are ongoing processes, and that feedback and setbacks are valuable tools for development.

Fixed or Growth Mindset?

First of all, let me ask you a question.

Do you think you have a Fixed or a Growth mindset?

Actually, we can be a bit of both.

Take the Quiz below to find out which way you lean.......

Fixed or Growth Mindset Quiz

Discover your mindset and how it influences your ability to grow and adapt. Answer the following questions honestly. For each statement, choose whether you agree or disagree.

1. **Intelligence is something you are born with, and it can't be changed.**
   o Agree
   o Disagree
2. **Challenges help me learn and grow.**
   o Agree
   o Disagree
3. **I prefer to avoid tasks that I might fail at.**

- o Agree
- o Disagree

4. **My abilities are set, and effort won't make much of a difference.**
   - o Agree
   - o Disagree

5. **When faced with a setback, I look for what I can learn from it.**
   - o Agree
   - o Disagree

6. **I often think, "I'm just not good at this," and leave it at   that.**
   - o Agree
   - o Disagree

7. **Success is about trying hard, not necessarily about being the best.**
   - o Agree
   - o Disagree

8. **If I don't succeed right away, I tend to lose motivation.**
   - o Agree
   - o Disagree

9. **Feedback helps me get better, even if it's critical.**
   - o Agree
   - o Disagree

10. **Talent alone determines success.**
    - o Agree
    - o Disagree

Scoring Your Results:

Count the number of times you answered "Agree" and "Disagree."

- **Mostly "Agree":** You lean towards a **Fixed Mindset**. This means you may see abilities as unchangeable. Reflecting on this mindset is a key first step towards unlocking new ways of learning and growing.
- **Mostly "Disagree":** You have a **Growth Mindset**. You likely believe that effort, perseverance, and learning from feedback can help you grow. This mindset can help you face challenges with resilience.

The Impact of a Fixed Mindset on Brain Health and Success

A fixed mindset can have several adverse effects on both brain health and success:

People with a fixed mindset tend to avoid challenges due to fear of failure. They believe that struggling with a task is a sign of inadequacy, so they stick to what they know and avoid anything that might expose their perceived weaknesses. This avoidance can result in low levels of mental stimulation, which is detrimental to brain health and can prevent the development of new neural connections.

Giving Up Easily: Those with a fixed mindset are more likely to give up when faced with obstacles. They see difficulties as insurmountable barriers rather than opportunities to learn and grow. This can result in a lack of resilience and weakening neural pathways associated with problem-solving and perseverance.

Ignoring Feedback: In a fixed mindset, feedback is often viewed as a personal attack rather than constructive criticism. People may ignore or reject feedback that could help them improve, missing out on opportunities to enhance their skills and abilities. This reluctance to accept feedback can hinder personal and professional growth.

Feeling Threatened by Others' Success: A person with a fixed mindset is more likely to feel threatened by others' success. They may feel a sense of inadequacy when others succeed. Rather than being inspired or learning from others' achievements, those with a fixed mindset may feel threatened, leading to negative emotions and lower self-esteem. This emotional stress can impact brain health, leading to anxiety and a lack of motivation.

Low Self-Esteem: Because a fixed mindset is rooted in the belief that abilities are innate and unchangeable, failure is often seen as a reflection of one's worth. This can lead to low self-esteem, as individuals may internalise failures and view them as evidence of their limitations rather than as opportunities to grow.

The Impact of a Growth Mindset on Brain Health and Success

A growth mindset, on the other hand, can significantly enhance both brain health and success.

People with a growth mindset seek out challenges, viewing them as opportunities to learn and grow. They are more prone to stepping outside of their comfort zone, which stimulates the brain, enhancing neuroplasticity and the creation of new neural connections. This can lead to greater cognitive abilities and mental resilience.

Persistence in the Face of Obstacles: A growth mindset encourages persistence, even when the going gets tough. By viewing obstacles as learning opportunities, individuals will likely stay motivated and persevere with their goals. This persistence strengthens the brain's problem-solving pathways and builds resilience.

Seeking Feedback: People with a growth mindset actively seek feedback, seeing it as an essential part of the learning process. By embracing constructive criticism, they can refine their skills and improve their performance. This openness to feedback helps create a feedback loop in the brain that reinforces positive behaviours and learning.

Learning from Others' Success: Instead of feeling threatened by others' achievements, people with a growth mindset are inspired and motivated by them. They seek to learn from others' successes, which can provide new insights and strategies for personal growth. This positive approach fosters community and collaboration, which benefits mental and emotional health.

High Self-Esteem: A growth mindset is associated with higher self-esteem because it is based on the belief that effort and learning lead to improvement. Failures are seen as temporary setbacks rather than defining moments, and individuals are more likely to view themselves as capable and resilient. Having this positive self-image contributes to overall well-being and mental health.

Cultivating a Growth Mindset

Adopting a growth mindset is more than changing your beliefs; it involves actively reshaping how you think and respond to challenges.

Ways to cultivate a growth mindset:

- **Change Your Self-Talk**: Listen to your language when talking to yourself. Replace negative, fixed mindset statements like "I can't do this" or "I'm just not good at this" with growth-oriented phrases like "I can learn how to do this" or "I'm getting better every day." This simple shift in language can change how you perceive your abilities and approach challenges.

- **Adopt a Positive Attitude**: Embrace the idea that barriers can be challenges that lead to opportunities for growth rather than threats to your self-worth. Focus on the process of learning and improvement rather than on the outcome. A positive attitude will help you stay motivated and resilient in facing difficulties.

- **Get Real & Be Specific**: Break down larger goals into smaller, achievable steps. This approach allows you to track progress and celebrate small wins, reinforcing your growth mindset. By setting specific goals, you can focus on the process of learning and improvement.

- **Celebrate Your Progress**: Take time to acknowledge and celebrate your efforts and progress, no matter how small. Recognising your achievements reinforces the belief that you can grow and improve, further strengthening your growth mindset.

By cultivating a growth mindset, you can enhance your brain health, build resilience, and unlock your potential for success. Remember, your brain is adaptable, and with the right mindset, you can continuously learn, grow, and achieve your desired outcomes.

What This Means for You

Your mindset plays a critical role in how you approach challenges, learning opportunities, and growth. Remember that the brain can change and grow if you lean more towards a fixed mindset. Shifting your perspective can open doors to new possibilities and more tremendous success.

Consider focusing on practices that reinforce a growth mindset - such as celebrating effort over outcomes, seeing challenges as learning opportunities, and recognising that skills can be cultivated over time. Next time you face an obstacle that slows down your progress or gives you an excuse to stop, try the following actions:

- Reflect on how this task supports your long-term goal
- Reflect on your intrinsic motivation
- Acknowledge your weaknesses and give

yourself a break by understanding that growth is a process. Ask yourself who do you know who that has already achieved what you want or has the skills you are working towards attaining. You do not have to reinvent the wheel!

- Change your language. Instead of saying or thinking, "I'm no good at this!" or "I failed!" say, "This is harder than I thought, but I can learn from this." Or "This is just a temporary obstacle to my long-term goal, and I can find a way around it."

A GROWTH MINDSET IN ACTION

On 25/10/2021, I gained my Brain Health Professional certification through Dr. Daniel Amen's 'Amen University' and became a Certified Brain Health Practitioner and Dr. Amen Licensed Brain Health Trainer. This gave me access to cutting-edge neuroscience tools and knowledge to assist individuals in reaching their true potential and peak performance.

In addition to my lived experience with severe traumatic brain injury, becoming an expert 'barrier-cracker' to overcome seemingly insurmountable obstacles, and working in the occupational rehabilitation industry for 18 years, this additional brain training enabled me to expand my knowledge and my business, to assist more individuals in overcoming their limiting beliefs.

'Molly' is the mother of a child who suffered an acquired brain injury when he was just a baby as a result of a bacterial infection.

She was advised on multiple occasions that she just had to adapt her son's life and her expectations and that her son would have limited opportunities due to his brain injury. She was left with little hope, but she did not allow the fixed mindset of some medical professionals to stop her from seeking solutions.

Molly saw my story of overcoming a severe traumatic brain injury to live a fulfilling and successful life via a podcast I had been invited to speak on. She reached out.

I began working with her son, starting with a Brain Optimisation Assessment to identify which areas of his brain required support.

I worked holistically with this young man and developed a brain optimisation plan based on his unique brain needs. At the time, he was experiencing severe anxiety, depression, memory and focus issues, self-esteem issues, and was socially isolated. He had experienced bullying through much of his school life and was unsure about his future, but he knew he wanted to be independent. This was his goal. He was on a government-funded Disability

Support Pension when we met, and he was doing some voluntary work but did not have any paid employment.

The initial stages of his brain-change program involved creating a brain-healthy lifestyle and changing his limiting beliefs.

Strategies within his Get Brain Fit! brain-change program included diet changes, exercise, brain training, a vocational assessment, neuro-linguistic programming (NLP) coaching, supplements to assist in balancing his brain, vocational study, mentoring, and anxiety relief hypnotherapy.

Today, that young man is thriving in life! His confidence has increased significantly! He runs Meetup groups, has many friends, and has a highly active social life. His IQ test scores have improved, plus he is working close to full-time, in paid employment in a role he loves. His mental and physical health has improved, and his future looks bright!

Brains CAN change.

Here are some scenarios of everyday life examples of how a mind can be in a growth or fixed state:

1. **Learning a New Skill**

- Sarah has always struggled with cooking, but she decided to take a cooking class. Even when she makes mistakes, she sees them as opportunities to improve. She believes that with practice, she'll improve and eventually master more complex dishes.

- Tori tries cooking once, burns the meal, and quickly gives up. She tells herself, *"I'm just not good at cooking,"* and avoids trying again.

2. **Receiving Feedback at Work**

- David gets constructive feedback from his boss about improving his presentation skills. He takes the advice seriously and works on improving, seeing feedback as a chance to grow and develop new skills.

- Tony receives feedback on a project but feels discouraged and defensive. He tries to justify his position and doesn't put effort into improving.

3. **Dealing with a Fitness Challenge**

- Maria is trying to get in shape but finds running difficult. Instead of quitting, she views the challenge as part of the process and sets small, achievable goals to improve her endurance.

- Tom tries running for the first time, finds it too exhausting, and quickly decides that he's "just not built for running." He is convinced that he'll never be able to get better, no matter what he does.

Did you pick the Growth and Fixed mindsets? Sarah, David, and Maria demonstrated Growth mindsets, while Tori, Tony, and Tom were examples of Fixed mindsets.

CHAPTER 4: The Chemistry of Joy

Serotonin is a chemical in the brain that helps control mood, emotions, and some body functions. It's often called the "feel-good" chemical because it makes people feel happy and well. Here's how serotonin affects your mood and ability to think flexibly:

1. **Mood Control**

Serotonin helps keep your mood steady. When you have the right amount, you feel calm, happy, and emotionally balanced. If you have too little, you might feel depressed, anxious, or easily upset. Some antidepressant medicines, like Selective Serotonin Reuptake Inhibitors, (SSRIs), work by raising serotonin levels to improve mood. Too much serotonin can be harmful too and can lead to serotonin-syndrome which can be fatal. If you are also taking a prescribed SSRI medication, it is critical to talk to your prescribing doctor before increasing your serotonin with supplements or increasing your medication dosage.

2. **Flexible Thinking**

Serotonin also helps the brain stay flexible. It lets you adjust to new situations, switch tasks, and solve problems from different angles. With enough serotonin, you can handle stress better and make decisions more easily.

3. **Emotional Strength**
   Serotonin helps you manage stress and stay positive, even in tough times. It helps you control your emotions and prevent you from getting overwhelmed by negative feelings.

4. **Sleep Support**
   Serotonin is also needed to make melatonin, a hormone that controls your sleep. By helping you sleep well, serotonin boosts your mental clarity and energy, which further improves your mood and thinking.

In short, serotonin helps you feel emotionally stable, handle stress better, and stay flexible in your thinking. Keeping your serotonin levels balanced is important for overall mental health and brain function.

When a Lack of Serotonin Keeps You STUCK: A True Story

'Janie' suffered debilitating anxiety over many years. She was raised in a good, loving family, and she was a competent lady. A single mother of two girls, Janie constantly felt like she was letting everyone down - her employer, her children, and her partner, because she was often stuck at home, vomiting into the toilet and unable to fulfill her promises and commitments. Janie was living with chronic anxiety.

Over the years, Janie attended many psychologists and counsellors. She had received good advice on 'how to manage stress and anxiety symptoms.' Janie regularly practiced meditation and was doing mostly the right things for her brain, including exercising regularly, but anxiety was still ruling her life.

Nobody had ever looked at Janie's brain despite attending many different counsellors and psychologists. None of her allied health professionals had addressed her brain health.

Until she booked in with me.

Following a Get Brain Fit! Brain Optimisation Assessment, I was able to identify that Janie had traits of attention deficit disorder (Combined ADD). She had increased activity in her Anterior Cingulate Gyrus (ACG), Basal Ganglia (anxiety centre) and the Limbic area of her brain. The ACG helps our brains think and do things flexibly. A healthy ACG can move from task to task, from thought to thought, from action to different action without too much stress. However, when our ACG is overactive, we will likely resist change with vengeance (Amen, 2015).

Picture the person beating their head against the proverbial brick wall. These people are likely to try the same thing over and over and over again......they hate change!

So, Janie's brain was struggling with decision-making, impulse control, memory, planning, and organisation, and it was resisting change. All of this was making her hyper-focused on worry and highly anxious. Additionally, the emotional centre of her brain was overactive, so she found herself crying for no apparent reason, feeling emotionally unregulated, and snapping at her children too often.

This combination of brain issues resulted in Janie needing to juggle multiple balls in the air at a time to keep her dopamine levels up (excitement) but without the capacity to manage these multiple balls due to distraction, overwhelm, and anxiety. The Prefrontal Cortex (PFC) area of her brain was compromised due to her ADD. Even though Janie tried really hard to keep all her commitments and function at a high level, she ended up frequently letting down the people around her because the Boss of her brain was stuck in 'off duty' mode much of the time, her Cingulate Gyrus was acting like cement to keep her stuck in a cycle of anxiety. Janie's brain needed a rebalance and some updated wiring.

Have you ever met someone who is inherently negative? Their glass is most frequently 'half empty' rather than 'half full.' From a conversational perspective, talking to a person who does not see many options in life to improve their situation can feel quite draining. They hate change, and when you suggest change, they will likely give you a big "NO!" without room for compromise.

If you work with customers and want to move them to a better product or service, the 'glass half empty' customer will be hard to convince. If you are managing a team and are trying to implement change management strategies, this person will resist. Timing is everything!

With a balanced brain, individuals will be more open to change, more comfortable considering alternative options, and more willing to make the necessary changes.

Individuals with elevated ACG issues are likely to have low Serotonin levels in the brain

(Amen, 2015).

CHAPTER 5: Preparing Your Brain for Change

Imagine your brain as the control centre of a vast, interconnected network. The intricate balance of this remarkable organ influences every thought, every emotion, and every habit you form.

Preparing your brain for change is more than just a mindset shift - it's about understanding the physical and functional foundation of your brain and optimising it for success. In this chapter, we'll explore how a balanced brain lays the groundwork for building and sustaining good habits, and how a Brain Optimisation Assessment can be the key to unlocking your potential.

The Foundation of Change: A Balanced Brain

Before creating or maintaining new habits, it's essential to understand the importance of brain balance. The prefrontal cortex - responsible for decision-making, focus, and impulse control, must work in harmony with other parts of the brain, such as the limbic system, which manages emotions. A brain that is in balance enables clarity, motivation, and emotional stability, all of which are critical for successfully adopting new habits.

Research from Dr. Daniel Amen, a leading expert in brain health, highlights that the prefrontal cortex plays a crucial role in goal-oriented behaviour and impulse control (Amen, 2018). When the prefrontal cortex functions optimally, you are better equipped to make choices that align with your long-term goals rather than succumbing to immediate impulses. Conversely, an imbalanced brain can lead to procrastination, emotional reactivity, and difficulty maintaining focus - barriers that often derail our best intentions to create positive change.

A balanced brain also supports neuroplasticity, the brain's ability to rewire itself in response to new experiences. As discussed in Chapter 2, Neuroplasticity is essential for forming new habits. When your brain is balanced, it is more adaptable, open to new patterns, and can better consolidate those patterns into long-term behaviour (Doidge, 2015). Ensuring your brain is in an optimal state is the first step toward effective habit formation.

The Role of the Brain Optimisation Assessment

So, how do you know if your brain is balanced and ready for change?

This is where the Brain Optimisation Assessment comes in. The assessment comprehensively evaluates your brain's functioning, identifying areas that need support to bring your brain into balance. The insights gained from this assessment can be truly transformative, giving you a clear picture of which brain regions may be overactive or underactive, and how this impacts your daily behaviour.

For example, someone with an overactive ACG, like 'Janie' in Chapter 4, might struggle with repetitive thoughts, making it challenging to break old habits and embrace new ones. The Brain Optimisation Assessment can pinpoint these imbalances and offer targeted strategies, such as cognitive exercises, nutritional changes, and mindfulness techniques that promote healthier brain activity.

By understanding your unique brain profile, you can create a tailored plan that optimises your brain for change instead of relying solely on willpower, which often fails when the brain is out of balance. You can leverage strategies that align with your brain's functioning with your goals. This approach makes habit formation easier and more sustainable in the long term.

Creating and Maintaining Good Habits

The process of building good habits involves three key stages: cue, routine, and reward

(Duhigg, 2012). A balanced brain enhances each of these stages, making the process smoother and more effective:

• **Cue Recognition**: A well-balanced brain is more attuned to recognising the cues that trigger desired behaviours. For example, if you want to start a morning exercise routine, a balanced prefrontal cortex helps you recognise the cue, such as the alarm clock, as a signal to get moving, rather than an opportunity to hit the snooze button.

• **Routine Formation**: Routine formation requires consistency and focus. When your brain is balanced, your ability to stay committed to a new routine improves. The basal ganglia, which plays a role in habit formation, works more efficiently when supported by an optimized brain environment (Graybiel, 2008).

• **Reward Processing**: Rewards reinforce habits, and a balanced brain enhances your ability to experience positive emotions from these rewards. When dopamine pathways function well, you feel more motivated and satisfied by your progress, which encourages you to stick to new habits.

The Game-Changer: Awareness and Action

One of the most powerful aspects of preparing

your brain for change is the awareness that comes from understanding your own brain's unique needs. The Brain Optimisation Assessment provides this awareness, allowing you to take targeted action that brings about real change. Instead of feeling frustrated by repeated failed attempts to create new habits, you gain a roadmap to understanding why these attempts may have faltered in the past and how to set yourself up for success moving forward.

Preparing your brain for change is not about perfection - it's about progress. It's about understanding that your brain's balance is the foundation upon which all good habits are built. By optimising your brain, you lay the groundwork for lasting transformation, empowering yourself to create the life you desire, one habit at a time.

The Get Brain Fit! Brain Optimisation assessment includes a comprehensive checklist of brain behaviours which you rate yourself against. When you have completed the assessment and hit the 'submit' button, your assessment results are analysed and you will receive an invite to book a personalised brain health consultation to discuss your results and you will receive recommendations to optimise your brain.

For more information, you can go to:
https://optimisemybrain.getbrainfit.com.au

Practical Strategies to Improve Brain Health and Unlock Your Full Potential

Strategy 1: Eat a Plant-Based Diet Rich in Antioxidants and Omega-3 Fatty Acids

Why It Works: A plant-based diet rich in antioxidants and omega-3 fatty acids have been shown to support brain health and cognitive function. Antioxidants help protect the brain from oxidative stress, which can lead to cellular damage and cognitive decline. Omega-3 fatty acids, particularly those found in fatty fish, such as salmon, are essential for maintaining the health of brain cells and promoting neuroplasticity.

Flaxseeds and Chia seeds are also great sources of Omega-3. However, because our bodies need to convert Alpha-linolenic acid (ALA) into Eicosapentaenoic acid (EPA) and Docosahexaenoic acid (DHA), and this conversion isn't very efficient, they shouldn't be your only Omega-3 intake.

Our diets have drastically changed from those of the early 1900's. Back then, fast food didn't exist, and highly processed products packed with salt, sugar, and Omega-6 fatty acids were not staples in our meals.

Even if you prepare your own meals at home, the quality of ingredients has unfortunately declined. Much of the meat we consume now comes from animals raised indoors on feed rather than grazing on grass in open fields. Similarly, fish like salmon are often farmed in controlled environments and fed fishmeal, rather than consuming algae in their natural deep-sea habitats. These changes significantly impact the nutritional value of our food, and by extension, the health of our cells, tissues, and overall well-being.

Understanding the Omega-6 to Omega-3 Ratio

Both Omega-3 and Omega-6 fatty acids are essential in our diet, but maintaining the right balance between the two is crucial. Unfortunately, 95% of people are at risk of having an imbalanced ratio. Without Omega-3 supplementation, many people can have a ratio as high as 25:1, far from the recommended balance (Clayton 2019).

The science is clear: for optimal health, a 3:1 ratio of Omega-6 to Omega-3 is ideal. However, many of us do not consume enough Omega-3's in our diet, leading to potential health risks. Rebalancing this ratio can significantly improve your overall health and well-being.

How to Implement It:

- Incorporate more fruits and vegetables into your daily meals, focusing on those high in antioxidants, such as berries, leafy greens, and cruciferous vegetables like broccoli and brussels sprouts.
- Include Omega-3-rich foods in your diet regularly. If you're not a fan of fish, consider adding flaxseeds, chia seeds, walnuts, and algae-based supplements such as spirulina, Nori, wakama, or kombu seaweed.
- Limit processed foods and foods high in saturated fats, which can negatively affect brain health over time.
- Consider adopting a Mediterranean-style diet. This diet is rich in plant-based foods, healthy fats, and lean proteins and has been linked to improved cognitive function and reduced risk of neurodegenerative diseases.

Other Diet Considerations

Your brain is your most important asset, and what you feed it matters.

Fresh fruits and vegetables are packed with essential nutrients, antioxidants, and fibre that nourish your brain and protect it from damage.

Unlike processed foods, which are often high in unhealthy fats, additives, and processed sugars, fresh produce supports your brain's ability to thrive.

Reducing processed sugar intake is especially critical. High sugar consumption can trigger inflammation and contribute to brain shrinkage over time, which impacts memory, focus, and mood. On the other hand, natural sugars from fruits provide energy alongside vitamins and minerals without the inflammatory effects of their processed counterparts.

By choosing fresh, whole foods over processed options, you not only protect your brain from harm but also fuel it to perform at its peak. Start small: swap a sugary snack for a colourful fruit salad or add a vibrant mix of veggies to your plate. Your brain will thank you!

Strategy 2: Engage in Regular Physical Exercise

Why It Works:

Exercise is one of the most effective ways to enhance brain health, and a critical factor in this process is Brain-Derived Neurotrophic Factor (BDNF). BDNF is a protein that plays a key role in neuroplasticity, which is the brain's ability to form new neural connections.

It helps support the survival of existing neurons and encourages the growth of new ones, which is crucial for learning, memory, and cognitive function.

When you engage in regular physical activity - especially aerobic exercise like running, cycling, or swimming—your body increases the production of BDNF. This, in turn, promotes the formation of new neural connections, improving overall brain health. High levels of BDNF have been linked to enhanced cognitive function, protection against neurodegenerative diseases, and even mood regulation (Douyon, 2018).

Here's how exercise and BDNF can benefit your brain:

- **Improved Memory:** BDNF enhances hippocampal function, the brain region responsible for memory and learning.
- **Increased Neuroplasticity:** By boosting BDNF levels, exercise helps your brain adapt and reorganize itself, which is essential for learning new skills or recovering from brain injury.
- **Mood Regulation:** BDNF also plays a role in reducing symptoms of depression and anxiety by promoting resilience in brain pathways linked to emotion regulation.
- **Protection Against Neurodegeneration:**

Higher BDNF levels help protect the brain from age-related diseases like Alzheimer's and Parkinson's.

Regular exercise, combined with proper nutrition and mental stimulation, offers a powerful way to boost BDNF levels and keep your brain healthy, resilient, and sharp.

How to Implement It:

- Incorporate aerobic exercises such as walking, running, swimming, or cycling into your routine, aiming for at least 150 minutes of moderate-intensity weekly exercise.
- Break this down into daily aerobic exercise of ideally 30 minutes per day, five days per week.
- Add strength training exercises like weightlifting or resistance band workouts to your routine at least twice weekly. Strength training has been shown to improve cognitive function, particularly in older adults.
- Include mind-body exercises like yoga, Pilates, or Tai Chi, which combine physical movement with mental focus and have been shown to reduce stress and improve cognitive function.

Strategy 3: Prioritise Quality Sleep

Why It Works: Sleep is critical for brain health because it is during sleep that the brain clears out toxins, consolidates memories, and repairs itself. Poor sleep has been linked to cognitive decline, memory problems, and increased risk of neurological disorders (Bredesen, 2020).

How to Implement It:

- Establish a regular sleep schedule by going to bed and waking up at the same time each day, even on weekends.
- Create a sleep-friendly environment by keeping your bedroom dark, cool, and quiet. Consider using blackout curtains, white noise machines, or earplugs if necessary.
- Avoid screens before bedtime. The blue light emitted by phones, tablets, and computers can interfere with your body's natural sleep-wake cycle. Try to limit screen time to at least an hour before bed.
- Practice relaxation techniques before bed, such as deep breathing, meditation, or reading a book, to help calm your mind and prepare your brain for restful sleep.

Strategy 4: Challenge Your Brain with New Learning

Why It Works: Engaging in new learning and mentally stimulating activities promotes neuroplasticity and helps build cognitive reserve, which is the brain's ability to adapt and compensate for changes or damage. Learning new skills or hobbies keeps the brain active and sharp.

How to Implement It:

- Take up a new hobby or learn a new skill that challenges your brain, such as playing a musical instrument, learning a new language, or taking up a creative art like painting or writing.
- Engage in puzzles and brain games that stimulate cognitive function, such as crosswords, Sudoku, chess, or memory games. These activities can improve problem-solving skills, memory, and focus. Remember to switch up your games because once you have become knowledgeable in how to do Sudoku or any other game, and it becomes pretty easy, you are getting less benefits to the brain. The brain thrives on novelty and challenge!
- Try out different cognitive exercises targeting other areas of the brain. For example, practice mindfulness meditation to enhance focus and emotional regulation, or engage in activities that require complex problem-solving to boost executive function.

Remember it is the 'new learning' path that challenges your brain and stimulates new neural pathways. If you keep repeating the same game or have mastered the language or musical instrument, you maintain that pathway, not build new ones. The message here is to keep your brain stimulated with continual learning.

Strategy 5: Cultivate Strong Social Connections

Why It Works: Social interaction is crucial for maintaining brain health. Engaging with others helps reduce stress, improve mood, and stimulate cognitive function. Having strong social connections has been strongly linked to a reduction in the risk of cognitive decline and dementia (Bredesen, 2017).

How to Implement It:
• Make time for social activities you enjoy, such as joining a club, participating in group fitness classes, or attending community events.
• Stay connected with family and friends by planning regular phone calls, video chats, or face-to-face visits. Meaningful conversations and shared experiences can strengthen your emotional well-being and cognitive function.
• Volunteering or participating in community service often provides a sense of purpose, can increase one's social network, and can benefit one's brain health.
• Consider joining online communities or social networks that align with your interests. Engaging in discussions, sharing ideas, and learning from others can stimulate your brain.

Bringing these strategies into your daily life will enable you to improve your brain health, enhance cognitive function, and unlock your full potential. These practices are scientifically supported but also practical and accessible, making them effective tools for optimising your brain and overall well-being.

BRAIN HEALTHY ACTIONS TO GET STARTED:

- ☐ Exercise for 30 minutes at least three times per week initially.
- ☐ Reduce consumption of processed sugar (table sugar, high-fructose corn syrup, artificial syrups etc)
- ☐ Get a minimum of 7 hours sleep per night.
- ☐ Minimise coffee and alcohol intake.
- ☐ Drink 2 litres of water every day.
- ☐ Start your day with gratitude practice – reflecting on what you are thankful for primes your brain for positivity and reduces stress!
- ☐ Focus on a diet rich in brain-boosting foods such as Omega-3 fatty acids and antioxidants (like salmon, sardines, walnuts, berries and leafy greens).
- ☐ Practice Mindfulness or Meditation: Dedicate 10-15 minutes daily as these practices reduce stress and enhance focus,

emotional control, and clarity.

- ☐ Connect with others: Building meaningful relationships is a powerful brain booster that enhances emotional and cognitive health.
- ☐ Limit screen time and protect our eyes: Set boundaries with technology to avoid overstimulation and enhance focus.
- ☐ Manage stress proactively: Use stress management techniques. Chronic stress can damage your brain!
- ☐ Laugh and Play: Make time for laughter, play, or humour every day! These activities reduce stress, improve creativity, and support brain resilience.
- ☐ Spend time outdoors: Natural sunlight supports Serotonin production.

Remember, you don't have to implement everything at once! Choose one new habit to implement each week and set yourself up for success.

CHAPTER 6: How Well Do You Know Your Brain?

Brain health experts have different ways of grouping brain types based on how we think, feel, and behave. Dr. Daniel Amen, my mentor and well-known brain specialist, created a framework with **five main core brain types** and 16 different brain types based on thousands of Single-Photon Emission Computed Tomography (SPECT) scans of the brain.

These brain types show how people's brains work and help explain why they react differently to the world around them.

In addition to the 16 different brain types, there are seven different types of attention deficit hyperactivity disorder (ADHD) and multiple types of anxiety and depression. It is vital to have as much information about your brain as possible to access the interventions that are going to work best for your unique brain.

A great example of this is a lady I worked with to assist with her return to work after experiencing severe depression and ADHD. She hadn't been able to function at work for over a year and was taking a cocktail of medications.

When I first met with 'Kim,' she advised that she felt like a "mouse on a wheel," getting nowhere.

Kim had been referred to a Psychologist and Psychiatrist and was attending regularly, but no one had looked at her brain!

She participated in a Get Brain Fit Brain Optimisation Assessment, and the areas of her brain that were suffering included her Pre-frontal Cortex (the Boss of the brain). She struggled with decision-making, planning, organisation, time management, focus and impulse control.

The area of her brain that allows for flexible thinking (Anterior Cingulate Gyrus) was also struggling, which meant she struggled with change and saw life through a 'glass half empty' lens. As you learned earlier, this area of the brain is important for emotional regulation, attention and focus, conflict detection and resolution.

Other areas of her brain which were suffering included the Limbic system (emotional brain) and Basal Ganglia (anxiety centre).

After reviewing her brain results and current prescribed medication, I could see there was a mismatch. The SSRI anti-depressant was slowing down her PFC function. Her PFC was already struggling due to her ADHD! This created the 'mouse on a wheel' effect. She needed a more stimulating anti-depressant.

Following consultation with her psychiatrist and his review of my Brain Optimisation Report, he changed her medication, and her symptoms improved to a point where she could return to work.

Looking at the brain can provide the missing piece of the puzzle to progress!

When 'Sally' contacted me, she told me about her diagnosis of ADHD. Sally was also on the Autism Spectrum. She really struggled to have conversations in crowded spaces. This caused her high anxiety, so she would avoid meeting people in busy venues wherever possible.

She was self-employed, and this fear limited her opportunities.

As we discussed her cognitive challenges,

including her inability to focus when there were loud noises around her, she shared that she felt "stupid" in crowded, noisy venues.

Following a Brain Optimisation Assessment, we identified that her brain showed traits consistent with issues across all brain systems. Her brain was seriously out of balance! She functioned on much less sleep than is recommended and struggled to focus on tasks that did not excite her.

As part of her brain-balancing activities, she learned to juggle, started taking specific supplements to balance her brain dysfunction, and made some changes to her diet and exercise regime based on her brain type.

It was about four weeks later that I got a phone call from Sally. This is a summary of what she said:

"Oh my God Nicole! You have changed my life! I can converse with anyone, ANYWHERE, and I don't feel stupid!"

This is an excellent example of how a brain can change at any age. Sally was in her mid-60s!

'Tom' has been on the same anti-depressant

medication for half a decade!

He struggled with brain fog, confusion, and low motivation and experienced challenges with maintaining focus. As an entrepreneur, this made his job more difficult as he was accountable for his service delivery and products.

Tom decided to have a Brain Optimisation Assessment. His responses to the questionnaire indicated traits of attention deficit disorder (without hyperactivity) consistent with Overfocussed ADD in addition to persistent symptoms of depression and an overactive ACG.

Following consultation with his General Practitioner, he decided to wean himself off his anti-depressants and substitute with lifestyle actions and supplements to boost his serotonin levels. (Note: this should only be done in consultation with medical advice).

A few weeks after implementing his new routine, he contacted me and said *"Nicole, I am feeling the best I have felt in years! I have more energy; I am more focussed and more motivated than I have felt in a very long time!"*

YES! Brains can change.

CHAPTER 7: Are You at the Cause or Effect of Your Brain?

Life is full of obstacles and challenges - there's no avoiding that. It's an ever-evolving dynamic that requires us to adapt and be flexible. However, how we respond to these challenges depends on whether we are living at the "Cause" or "Effect" of our lives. (James, T., & Woodsmall, W. 1988). This mindset shift can significantly influence our success in achieving our goals and how empowered or powerless we feel in our personal lives and businesses.

Would you like to feel more empowered? To enjoy more fulfillment and success in your life and business? If your answer is "yes" to any of these questions, it's time to discover how many options you have to actualise your desired future.

Living at the Effect of Your Brain & Your Life

Many people go through life at the "Effect" of their circumstances. When things don't go as planned - when obstacles arise - they find reasons or excuses, often blaming external factors or even themselves. Living at the Effect means letting life control you, rather than taking control. People who live at Effect often use language like:

- "I can't…"
- "He/she told me I wasn't ready yet…"
- "It's because of…"
- "It's just how things are…"
- "I've always been like that…"
- "I reacted that way because he said…"
- "It's not my fault…"

These statements are limiting and prevent progress. They keep individuals and businesses stuck and unable to move forward.

Living at the Cause of Life

On the other hand, people who live at the "Cause" of their lives take action. They take conscious responsibility for their feelings, choices, and actions. They are proactive and willing to try different solutions until they achieve their goals. Even if they cannot control everything around them—like the weather, other people's behaviour, or opinions—they take ownership of what they can control: their beliefs, actions, and mindset.

People who live at the Cause of their lives might say:

- "I am ready to…"
- "I am in control of what I get from life."

- "I am going to succeed despite…"
- "I create my own opportunities."
- "I can make my own choices."
- "I can do anything I put my mind to."
- "I was part of the cause of that happening."

Living at Cause is about focusing on solutions, whereas living at Effect is about focusing on problems.

A Journey from Effect to Cause

It's okay if you recognise some of the "Effect" phrases in your own language. I've been there too. It took me three years to contemplate and procrastinate over whether I was "smart enough" to go to university. It took me a year to realise that my lack of confidence was merely an excuse delaying a keynote presentation I was asked to give. Confidence doesn't come from thinking about doing something - it comes from doing it!

It also took me years to write my first book because I feared that disclosing my traumatic brain injury would lead to negative judgment from employers and peers, making it harder for me to find work. But by pushing through my fear and publishing my first book, Holding on to Hope, Finding the 'New You' after a Traumatic Brain Injury, I found myself more in demand than ever!

By taking control of my narrative - by living at Cause - I created new opportunities and found the success I was seeking.

Choosing to Live at Cause

If you're ready to change your mindset, step into empowerment, and start fulfilling your goals through a positive and proactive framework, I'd love to help you!

CHAPTER 8: The Steps to Your True Potential

Congratulations on reading this far!

How long does it take to change your brain?

The time it takes to change your brain can vary depending on several factors, such as the type of change, your consistency, and the methods used.

Generally, the concept of neuroplasticity - your brain's ability to adapt and change, allows significant changes to occur over weeks to months (Doidge, 2007).

The key is **consistency** - whether through mental rehearsal, meditation, other brain training, learning new skills, or some of the lifestyle changes already discussed. Small, daily efforts can lead to long-term, impactful changes in how the brain functions, ultimately leading to a healthier, more adaptive, and resilient mind.

Remember to consult your medical professionals before making any changes which may impact on your current medical diagnosis and medications.

I am going to take an educated guess here and presume that you would like to change something about your mindset, cognitive function, or emotional regulation!

It is time to start taking action!

Hopefully, the information in this book has taught you about some changes you may like to make to improve your brain health.

If you would like to start this process by working towards a balanced brain, you can go to:
https://optimisemybrain.getbrainfit.com.au to take the Brain Optimisation Assessment.

The Benefits of a Brain Optimisation Assessment

A Brain Optimisation Assessment is a powerful tool that helps you understand your brain's current state and discover ways to unlock its full potential. Examining key areas of brain function, it provides personalised insights into how you can enhance clarity, memory, mood, focus, and productivity.

✅ Boost your energy and cognitive

functioning.

✅ Enhance your mood, memory and mental agility. Build cognitive reserves.

✅ Reduce inflammation, slow brain aging, and reduce risks of neurodegeneration.

✅ Enhance your productivity and focus.

✅ Get greater self-awareness. The assessment helps you understand your strengths and areas for growth, empowering you to make changes that directly impact your success and well-being.

Now, it is time to find your FUEL and Get Ahead Strategies (GAS) to move toward your desired life outcomes.

What would you like to achieve in the next three months, the next six months, or the next year?

Now, if you are ready to put in the effort, let's start the process of making your desired outcomes happen!

Are you ready to create the FUEL to propel you towards your goal realisation?

Goals sound boring, like hard work. If you have ever tried to create SMART goals, you may have become disillusioned by the process and stopped there, or you may love SMART goals.

I am going to assume that you are not going to make unrealistic goals!

Thanks to discoveries in neuroscience, we know that our brains are highly visual, and approximately 80% of sensory information is processed visually. The brain prioritises visual information due to the large neural real estate dedicated to it. (Medina, 2012)

The Cognitive Clarity Framework: Build Bridges to Your Goals

F — Focus on what you want

U — Understand the Path

E — Eliminate the Obstacles

L — Light Up the Process!

The Get Brain Fit! way to help you clarify your vision, strategise effectively and create the mental resilience needed to succeed in your goals!

GET**Brain**FIT

Now, let's fuel your way towards clarity on your goals to bring them to life!

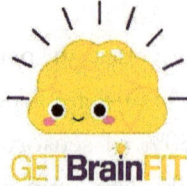

GET**Brain**FIT

The Cognitive Clarity Framework: Build Bridges to Your Goals

Step 1: Focus on What You Want (F - FUEL)
1. **Define Your Goal Clearly:**

   What is the specific outcome you want to achieve?

   (Example: "I want to launch my own online course by June 2025.")

   _____

   _____

2. **Why is this goal important to you?**
   (Example: "This will help me achieve financial independence and share my expertise.")

   _____

   _____

Step 2: Understand the Path (U - FUEL / Identify the Gap - BRIDGE)

- **Current Reality:**

  Where are you now in relation to this goal?
  (Example: "I have an idea for a course but no clear plan or resources.")

  _____

- **Desired Future:**

  What does success look like?
  (Example: "The course is live and generating $5,000 per month.")

  _____

- **Identify the Gap:**

  What key differences exist between your current reality and your desired future?
  (Example: "I lack a structured course outline and marketing plan.")

  _____

- **Brainstorm Paths:**

  List 3 possible ways to bridge this gap:

  1. _____

  —

  2. _____

  —

  3. _____

  —

Step 3: Eliminate Obstacles (E - FUEL)
1. **Anticipate Challenges:**

   What obstacles might block your progress?
   (Example: "Time constraints, lack of technical skills.")

   Your Obstacle #1:

   Obstacle 2:

   Obstacle 3:

2. **Brainstorm Solutions:**

   How will you overcome these obstacles? (Hint: what resources or strengths do you already have to help move you through these obstacles, including people you know who have already achieved this goal).

   List potential solutions for all obstacles:

   •

Step 5: Light Up the Process (L - FUEL / Anchor in the Why - BRIDGE)

Define Milestones (Define Milestones - BRIDGE)

1. **Small Wins:**

What smaller, measurable steps will help you track progress?
(Example: "Week 1: Draft course outline. Week 2: Record first module.")

Hint: Try inputting your goal into Goblin Tools to break it down! This AI resource is designed to simplify complex activities, automatically breaking down tasks into manageable steps.

2. **At What Points Will You Celebrate Success?**
(Example: "After completing the first module, celebrate with a weekend off.")

_____

_____

3. **Anchor in Your Why:**
What compelling reason will keep you motivated when the going gets tough?
(Example: "This course is my ticket to freedom and inspiring others.")

_____

4. **Visualise Success:**

Picture yourself achieving this goal. How will you feel?
(Example: "I'll feel proud, accomplished, and energised.")

_____

5. **Reward Yourself:**

What reward will you give yourself for reaching key milestones or the final goal?

(Example: "A holiday to celebrate the launch of the course.")

Step 6: Start Strong (Act Immediately – Get Ahead Strategy - GAS)

First Action Step:

What is the very first thing you will do to move closer to your goal today?
(Example: "Research online course platforms.")

Accountability:

Who can help keep you accountable, and how will you check in with them?
(Example: "I'll share my progress weekly with a mentor.")

Now, let's create your 'Grit-O-Meter'!

The 'Grit-O-Meter' is a Get Brain Fit! way to measure your current state of resilience and an easy visual cue to remind you of the things that will elevate your grit level (see next page).

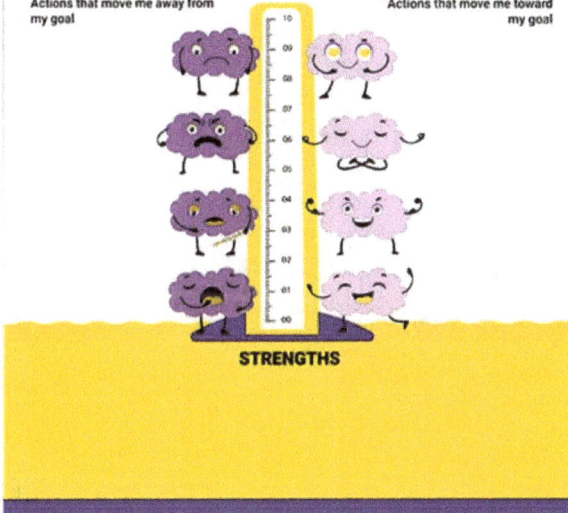

Grit-O-Meter

MY GOAL

YOUR GOAL
Actions that move me away from my goal

YOUR GOAL
Actions that move me toward my goal

10
09
08
07
06
05
04
03
02
01
00

STRENGTHS

It is now time to clarify your goal. State your goal as if you have already achieved it, and include a completion date. For example;

'By June 30, 2025, I have implemented a brain-healthy lifestyle that improves my memory, mood, and energy by consistently eating brain-supportive foods, exercising regularly, and practicing daily stress management techniques consistent with my unique brain needs'.

It is now time to measure your grit toward this goal.

Is this a goal you have tried before?

If you have tried your goal before and have not had the level of success you desired, that is okay. This process may help you identify the things that derailed your progress, and then you can develop strategies to avoid that derailment.

Looking at the Grit-o-Meter, where do you assess yourself as far as grit you have to reach this goal? Here is a scale to help you:

Grit-O-Meter Scale:

0. **Completely Given Up**: The person has tried to achieve the goal but has entirely given up. They feel there are no possible ways forward, and confidence is at its lowest point.

1. **Initial Re-Engagement**: The person is attempting again to move toward their goal, but with very low confidence. They are hesitant, and their belief in their ability to succeed is minimal.

2. **Slight Effort**: There is a small amount of effort being put forth. The person may feel some motivation but still lacks a strong sense of determination or direction.

3. **Occasional Attempt**: The person makes sporadic attempts toward their goal, possibly because they feel overwhelmed or do not see immediate progress. Their efforts are inconsistent.

4. **Some Commitment**: The person has shown more dedication. They have begun to set small, manageable steps but still struggle with self-doubt and occasional setbacks.

5. **Balanced Approach**: There is a mix of effort and belief. The person is actively working toward their goal but is not yet consistent. There are moments of strong drive but also times of struggle.

6. **Persistent but Struggling**: The person pushes through despite barriers and demonstrates resilience. They may face challenges, but their determination to keep trying is evident.

7. **Focused and Learning**: The person has developed a clearer strategy and learned from past mistakes. They consistently move forward, even when setbacks occur, showing strong resilience.

8. **Adapting and Growing**: The person has started finding different approaches when things don't work out. They are learning from each experience and adapting their strategies, growing stronger and more capable.

9. **Resilient and Innovative**: The person faces barriers head-on and finds creative solutions to overcome them. Their confidence is high, and they are making significant progress toward their goal.

10. **Unwavering Grit**: The person has overcome multiple barriers and has not given up. They have found ways around obstacles, gained new learnings, and continuously improved. They are very close to achieving their goal, and their confidence is unwavering.

This scale provides a comprehensive way for individuals to assess their current level of grit and understand how to move upward.

Next, write down all the current strengths and resources you already have to move you toward your goal. For example, you may have a Brain Optimisation Assessment report that gives you the roadmap to your goal, or you may have an exercise buddy or a gym membership. One of your strengths could be the meditation app you downloaded onto your phone or your intrinsic motivation for the goal outcome. Think of all your strengths and resources, including external and internal strengths.

Next, list all the actions you are currently doing

that move you toward your goal (on the right-hand side). Then, write down all of your current actions that move you away from your goal on the left-hand side of your Grit-o-meter. Some common progress delayers are hitting snooze instead of getting up in the morning, not scheduling the action/activity that moves you closer to your goal in your calendar and not setting reminders.

Before we get to your calendar, it is time to prioritise your activities and actions to help you achieve all aspects of your goal.

Introducing the Brain-Powered Action List:

GOALS FOR THE WEEK

TO DO LIST

01.
02.
03.
04.
05.
06.
07.
08.
09.
10.
11.
12.
13.
14.
15.

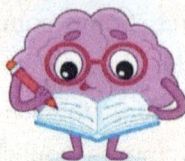

	URGENT	NOT URGENT
IMPORTANT	DO	SCHEDULE
NOT IMPORTANT	DELEGATE	DELETE

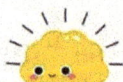

GET**Brain**FIT

List all the actions needed to propel you towards your goal.

I tend to spend up to 30 minutes on Sunday afternoon planning my next week, but some of my clients like to do this at the end of each day to prepare for the next day. Once you have brainstormed all of your 'To Do's, run them through the Eisenhower Matrix (Eisenhower, D.D. n.d) and allocate your resources and time accordingly. This framework helps individuals prioritise tasks based on urgency and importance and is widely attributed to President Dwight D. Eisenhower's productivity approach.

Green: Urgent and Important: This information is best scheduled in your calendar. If it is really important, and you are likely to get distracted or have time blindness, it can be a good idea to set your phone's clock alarm as a reminder for the urgent and important actions.

Orange: Urgent, but Not Important: Schedule it! These are activities that may be time-dependent and are important to do, but they are not urgent. These actions get scheduled in your Organiser, whether that is your Google Calendar or other scheduler.

Blue: Not Important, but Urgent: These are tasks that really should be delegated. If you have a Virtual Assistant, you could give them access to your email so they can respond to unimportant emails that require a response, for example. Or if you have unnecessary meetings that could be easily summarized via email because they don't require your direct input. What can you delegate to keep your focus on the important and urgent actions toward your goals?

Red: If they are not important and not urgent, then they need to be deleted. Examples of this may be responding to unnecessary emails or engaging in procrastination activities which only serve to help you avoid the more important tasks.

Now you are ready for action, to go forth and conquer your chosen goal!

It is time to celebrate your achievement by clarifying your goal and setting your brain-driven action plan!

Remember, it is important to reward yourself for each milestone you achieve toward your goal.

If you would like further support in working toward your goals, please don't hesitate to reach out. I love assisting people in reaching their true potential!

For more information, go to
https://www.getbrainfit.com.au

I would also love to offer you a free gift – the Get Brain Fit! 'How to Optimise Your Brain for Peak Performance Guide'

GET YOUR FREE GIFT!

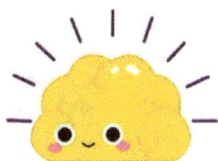

GETBrain**FIT**

freeguide.getbrainfit.com.au

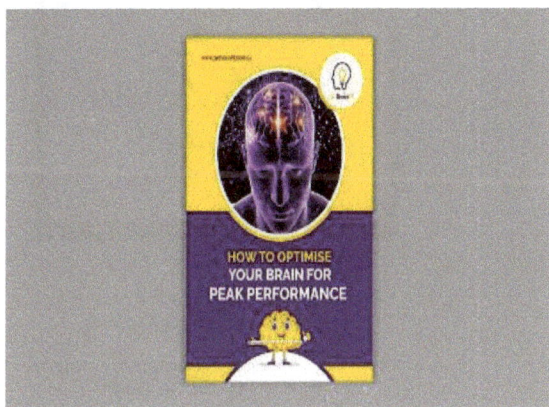

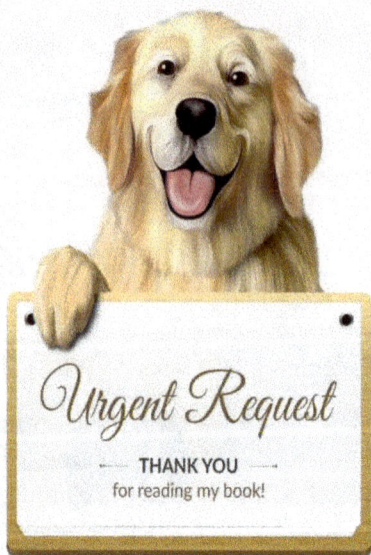

Urgent Request

— THANK YOU —
for reading my book!

I sincerely appreciate your feedback on my book, and I would love to hear what you have to say.

Please leave me a helpful review on Amazon letting me know what you thought of the book.

Thank you so much!

Nicole Yeates

References

- Alzheimer's Association. (2024). *Alzheimer's Disease Facts and Figures*. Alzheimer's Association. Retrieved 30.11.2024, from https://www.alz.org/alzheimers-dementia/facts-figures

- Amen Clinics. (n.d.). *How to slash your dementia risk by half*. Amen Clinics. Retrieved 02/12/2024, from https://www.amenclinics.com.

- Amen, D. (2018). *Change Your Brain, Change Your Life*. New York: Harmony Books.

- Bandler, R., & Grinder, J. (1979). *Frogs into Princes: Neuro Linguistic Programming*. Moab, UT: Real People Press.

- Bredesen, D. E. (2017). *The End of Alzheimer's: The First Program to Prevent and Reverse Cognitive Decline*. Penguin Random House.

- Bredesen, D. E. (2020). *The End of Alzheimer's Program: The First Protocol to Enhance Cognition and Reverse Decline at Any Age*. Penguin Random House.

- Clayton, P. (2019). *Complex inflammation*. Retrieved 02.12.2024, from https://drpaulclayton.eu/blog/complex-inflammation

- Costandi, M. (2016). *Neuroplasticity.*

Cambridge, MA: MIT Press.

- Doidge, N. (2007). *The Brain That Changes Itself: Stories of Personal Triumph from the Frontiers of Brain Science.* Viking Press.
- Doidge, N. (2015). *The Brain's Way of Healing: Remarkable Discoveries and Recoveries from the Frontiers of Neuroplasticity.* New York: Viking.
- Douyon, P. (2018). *Neuroplasticity: Your Brain's Superpower.* Izzard Ink.
- Duhigg, C. (2012). *The Power of Habit: Why We Do What We Do in Life and Business.* New York: Random House.
- Dweck, C. (2006). *Mindset: The New Psychology of Success.* Random House
- Graybiel, A. M. (2008). Habits, Rituals, and the Evaluative Brain. *Annual Review of Neuroscience*, 31, 359-387.
- Healthline. (2021). The Science of Habit: How to Rewire Your Brain. Retrieved from https://www.healthline.com/health/the-science-of-habit
- Huberman, A. (2021). The Science of Making & Breaking Habits. *Huberman Lab.* Retrieved from https://www.hubermanlab.com/episode/the-science-of-making-and-breaking-habits
- IBE–UNESCO. (n.d.). *Neuroplasticity: How the brain changes with learning.* Science of Learning Portal. Retrieved 02.12.2024, from https://solportal.ibe

unesco.org/articles/neuroplasticity-how-the-brain-changes-with-learning

- Integrative Psych. (2023). Decoding the Habit Loop: Unraveling the Neuroscience of Behavior Change. Retrieved from https://www.integrative-psych.org/resources/decoding-the-habit-loop-unraveling-the-neuroscience-of-behavior-change

- James, T., & Woodsmall, W. (1988). *Time Line Therapy and the Basis of Personality*. Cupertino, CA: Meta Publications.

- Livingston, G., et al. (2020). Dementia prevention, intervention, and care: 2020 report of the Lancet Commission. *The Lancet*,

- Medina, John. (2008) *Brain Rules: 12 Principles for Surviving and Thriving at Work, Home and School*

- Merzenich, M. M. (2013). *Soft-Wired: How the New Science of Brain Plasticity Can Change Your Life*. San Francisco: Parnassus Publishing.

- National Institute on Aging. (n.d.). *Alzheimer's disease genetics fact sheet*. U.S. Department of Health and Human Services. Retrieved 02.12.2024, from https://www.nia.nih.gov/health/alzheimers-causes-and-risk-factors/alzheimers-disease-genetics-fact-sheet

- Neurolaunch. (2023). Habit Formation in the Brain: Neuroscience Explained. Retrieved from https://neurolaunch.com/how-are-habits-formed-in-the-brain/

- Psychology Today. (n.d.). *Neuroplasticity*.

Retrieved 02/12/2024, from
https://www.psychologytoday.com/us/basics/neuroplasticity

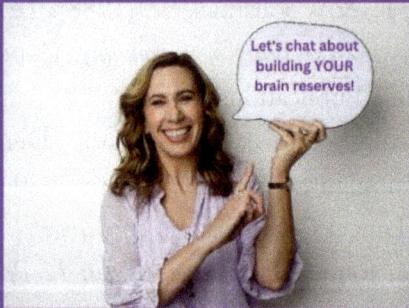

Phone: 0466 123 370
Email: nicole@getbrainfit.com.au

Find out more........
www.getbrainfit.com.au

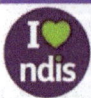

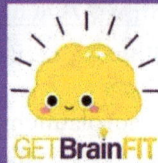